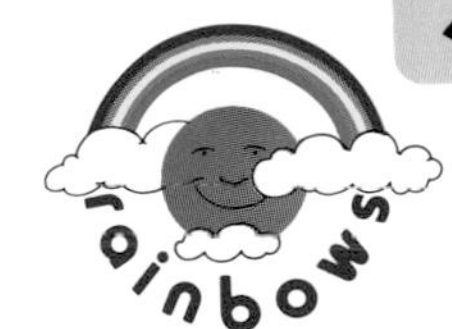

Look out at Home

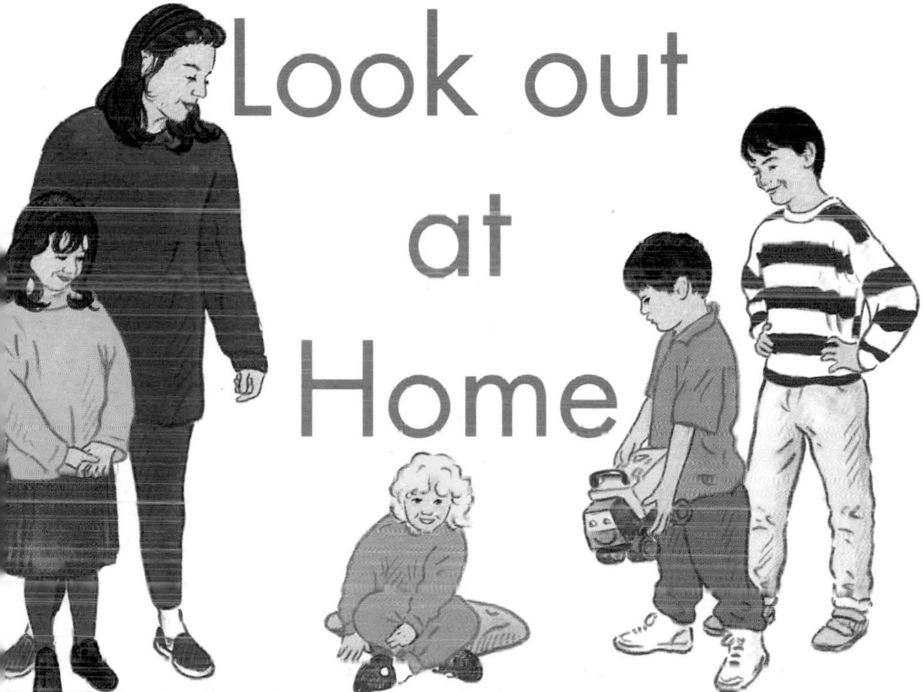

Helena Ramsay

Illustrated by

Derek Brazell

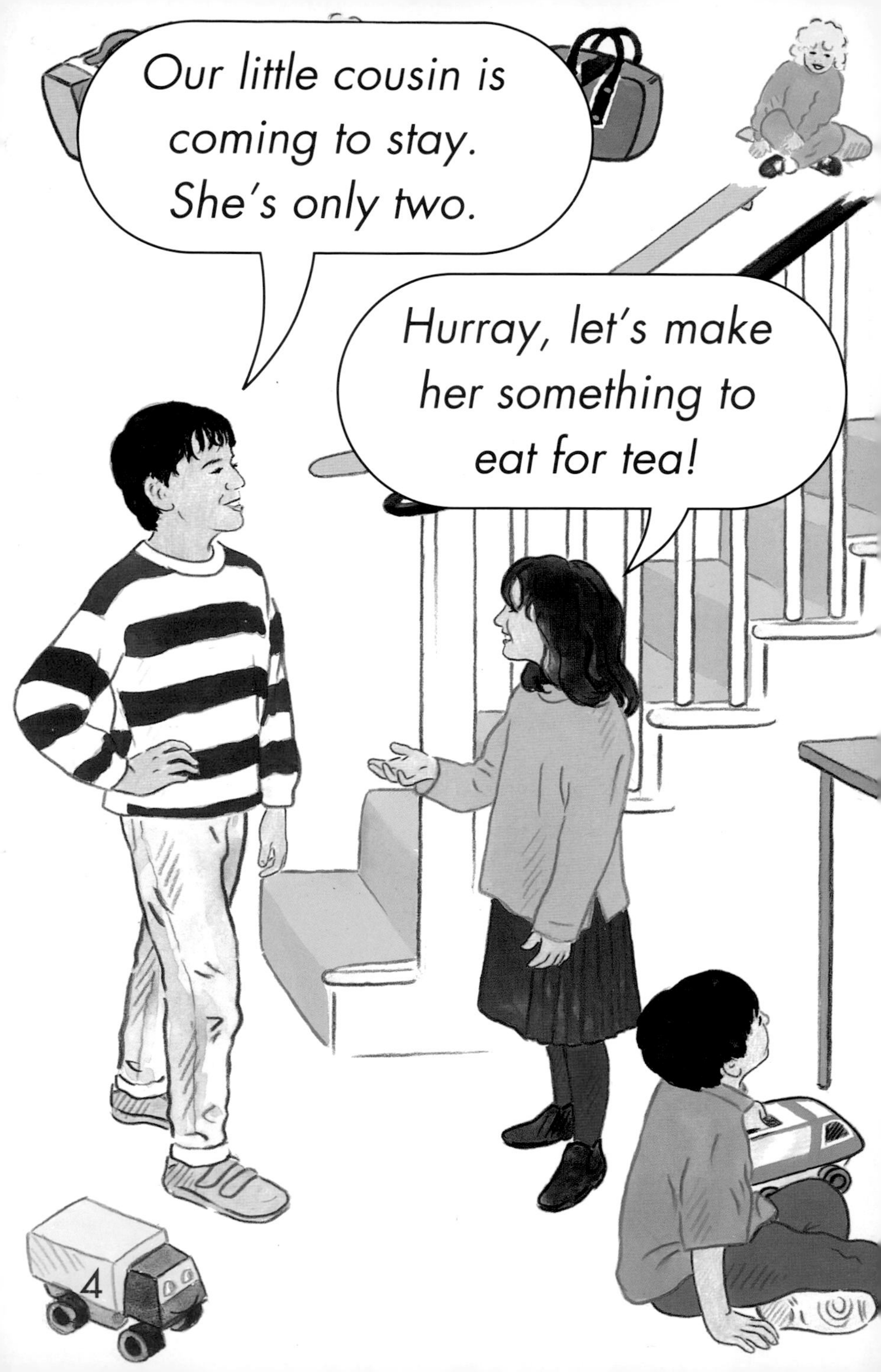
Our little cousin is coming to stay. She's only two.
Hurray, let's make her something to eat for tea!

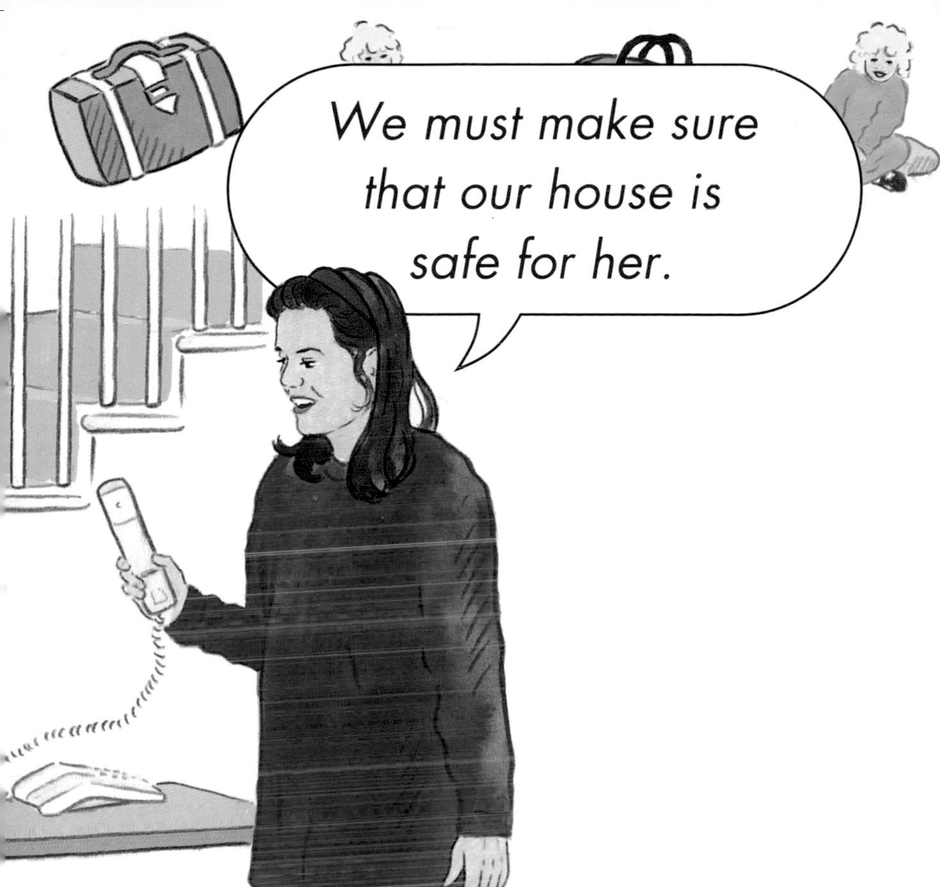

There are things in every house that can hurt babies and children like you. You have to be careful.

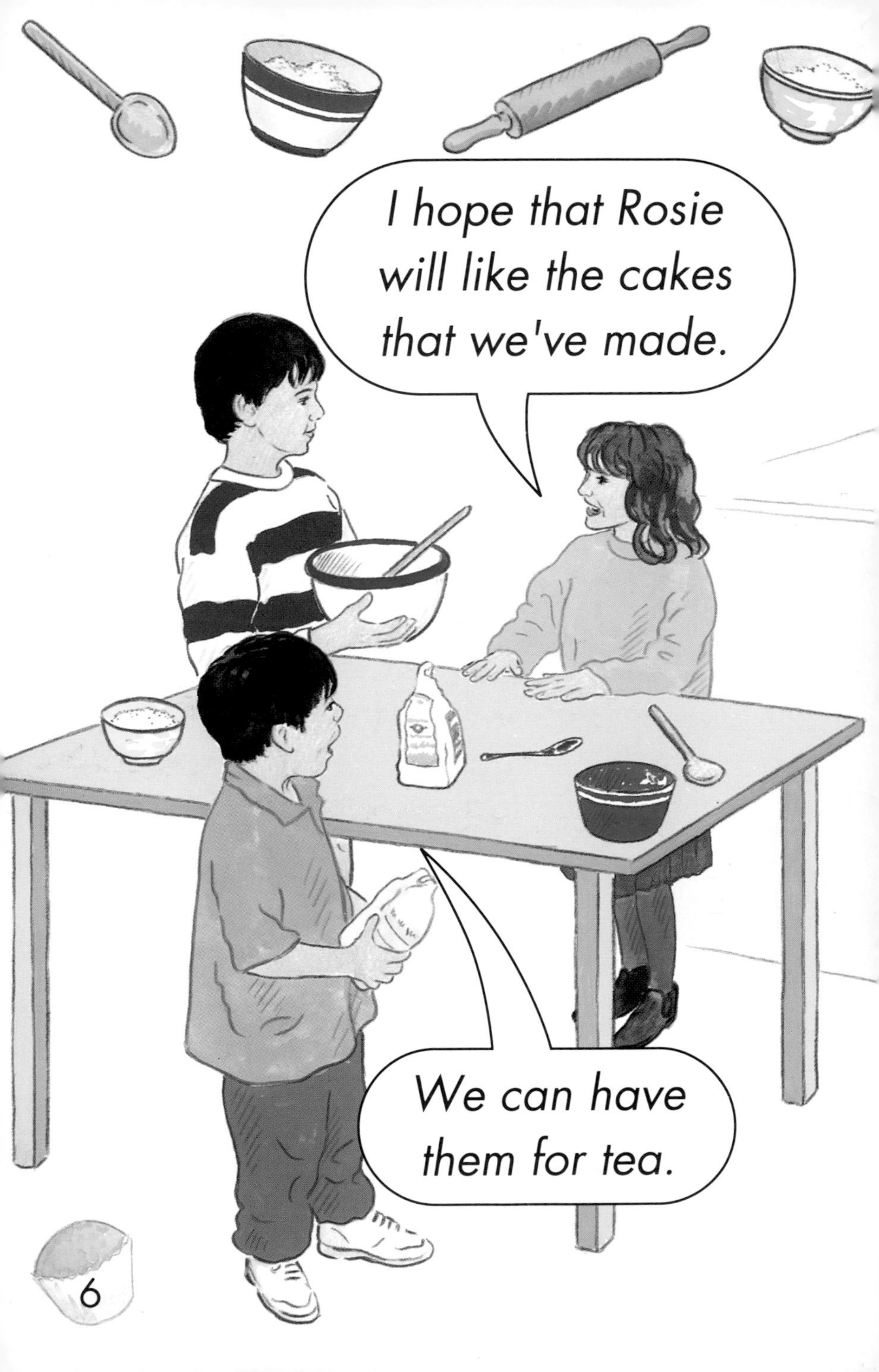
I hope that Rosie will like the cakes that we've made.
We can have them for tea.

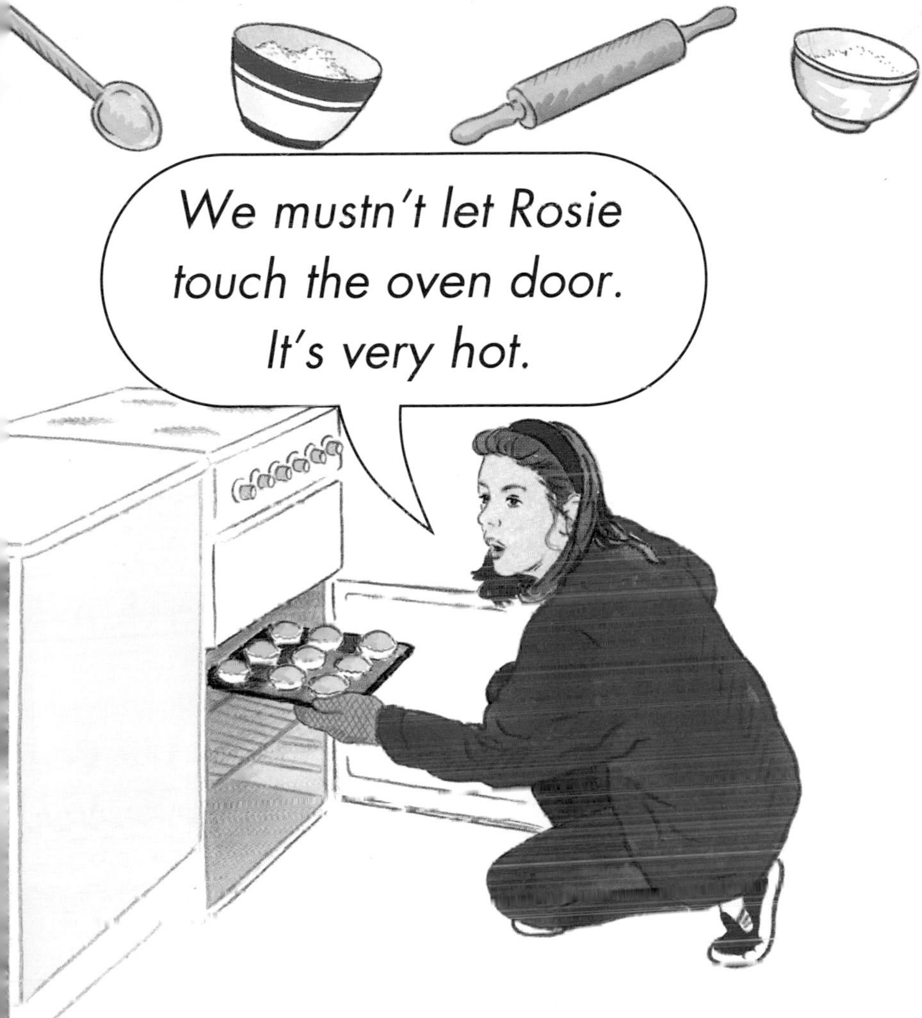

We mustn't let Rosie touch the oven door. It's very hot.

Never touch the cooker.
You could get burnt.

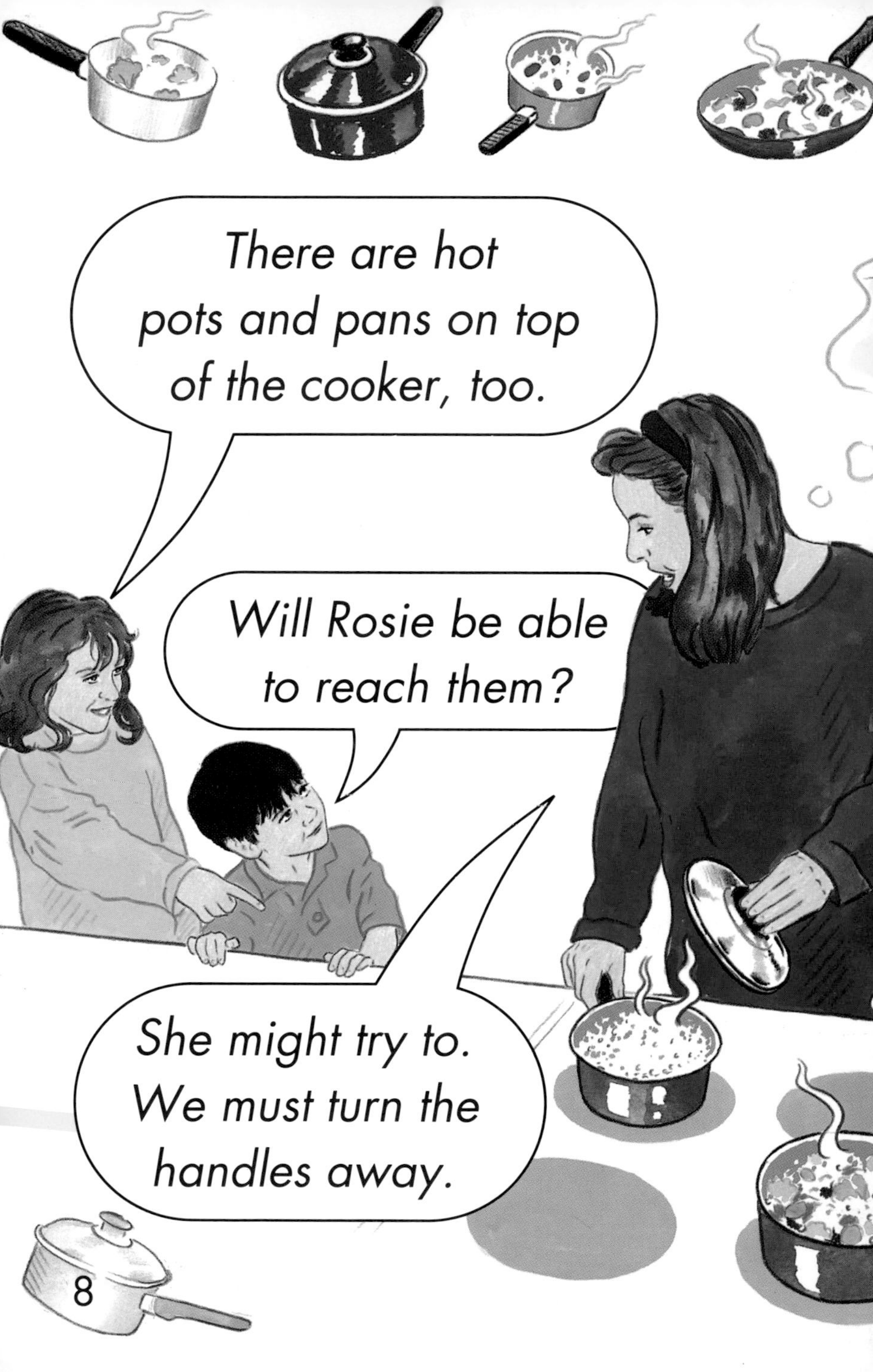
There are hot pots and pans on top of the cooker, too.
Will Rosie be able to reach them?
She might try to. We must turn the handles away.

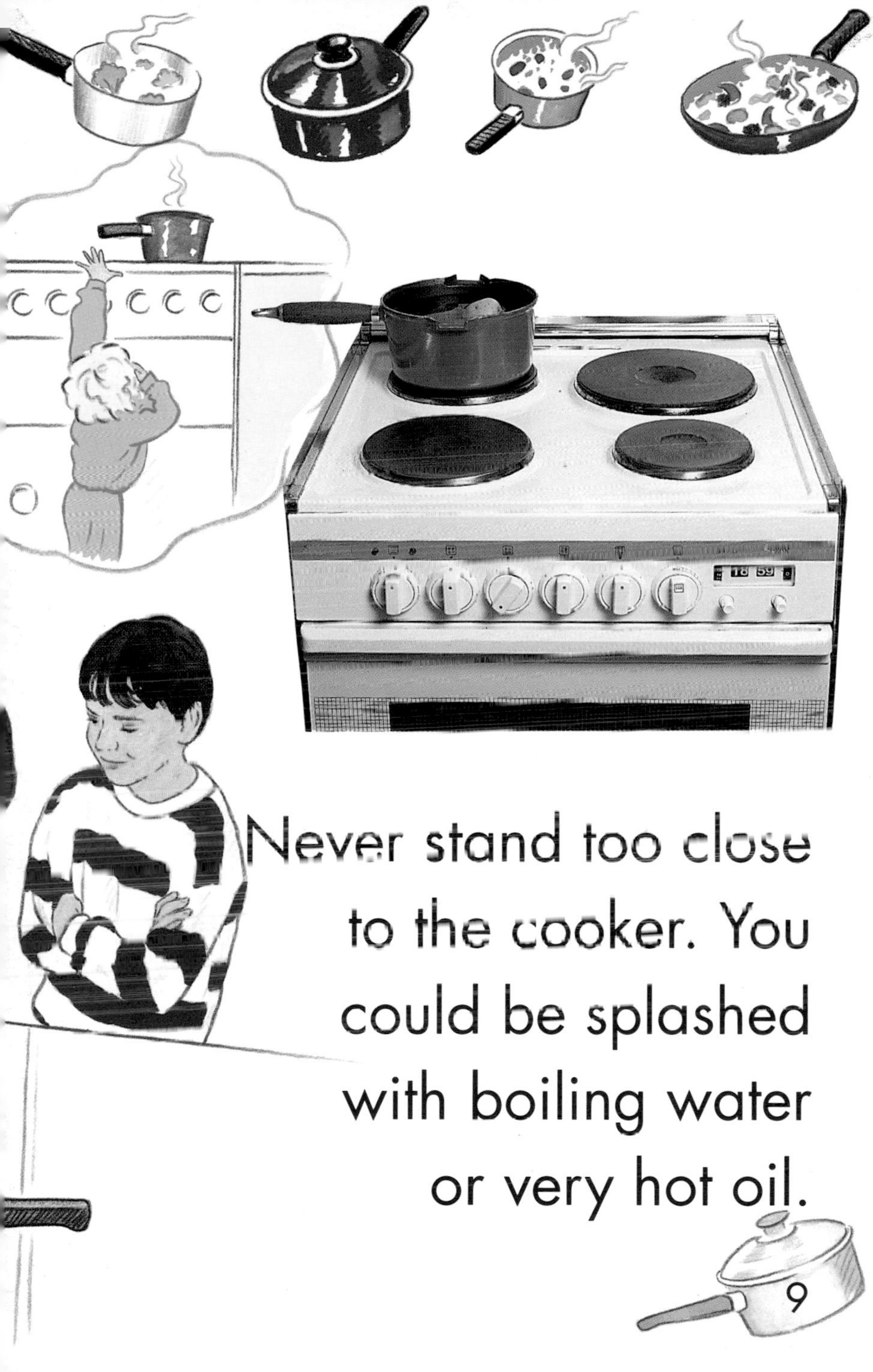

Never stand too close to the cooker. You could be splashed with boiling water or very hot oil.

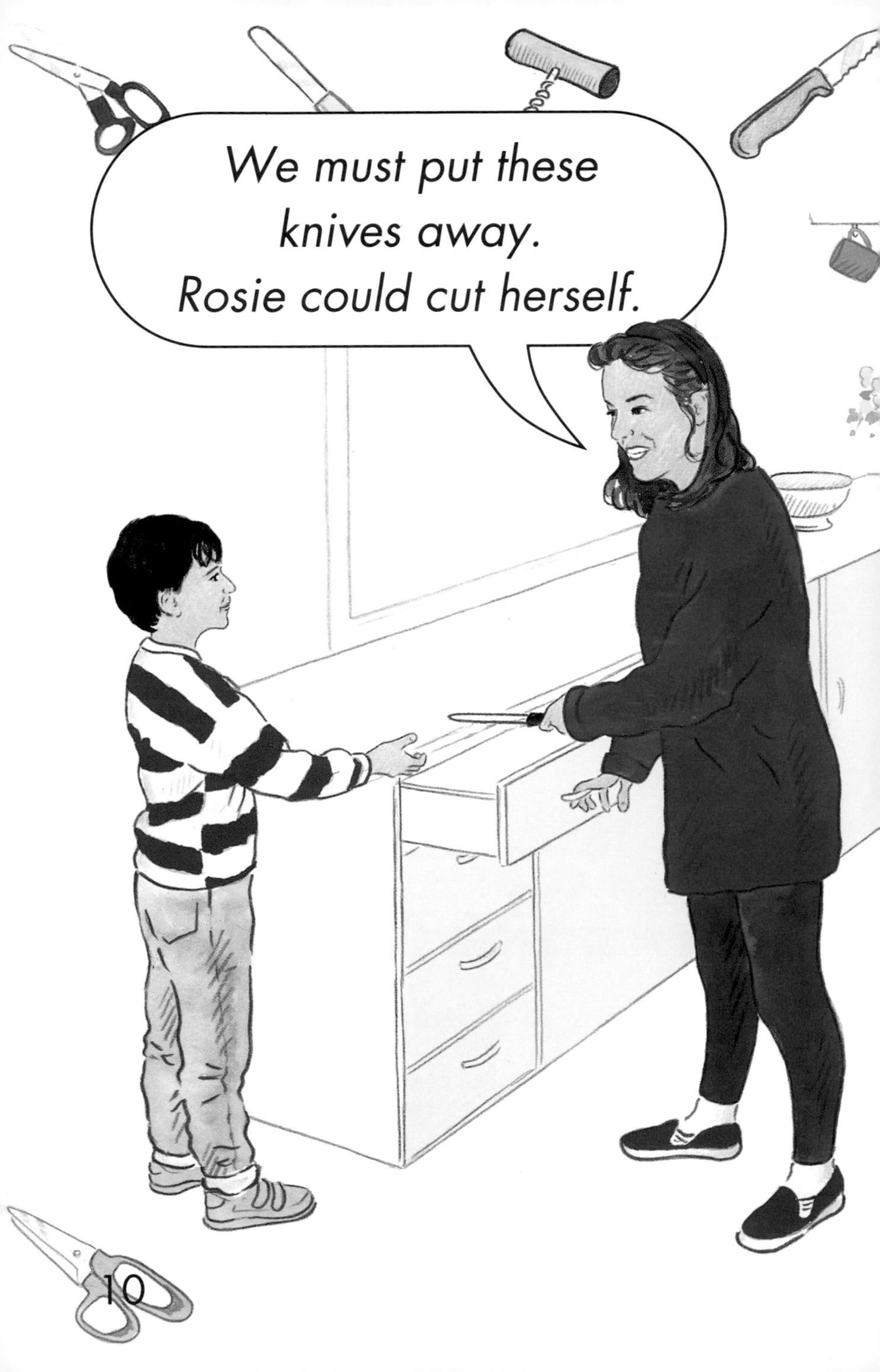
We must put these
knives away.
Rosie could cut herself.

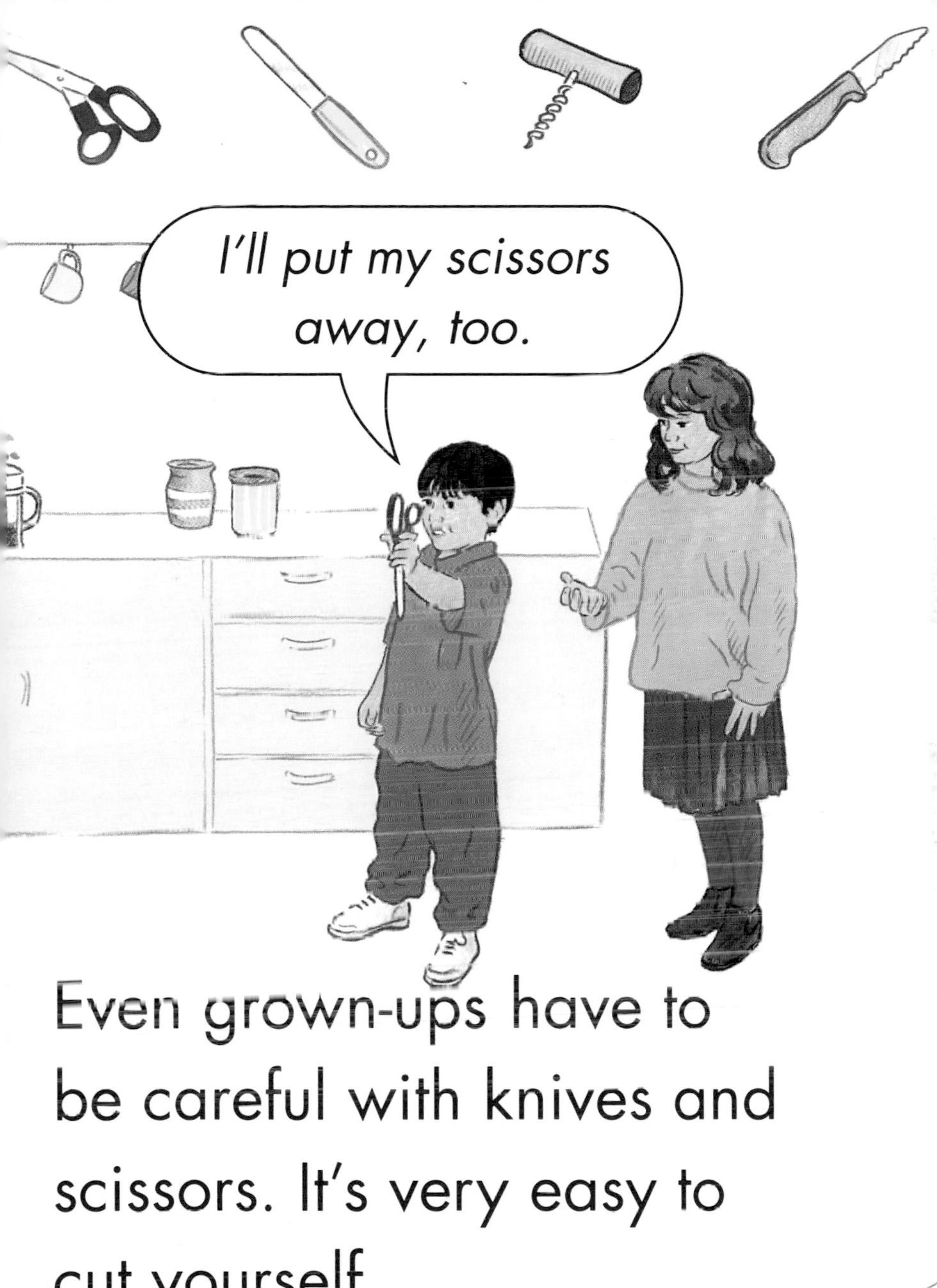

Even grown-ups have to be careful with knives and scissors. It's very easy to cut yourself.

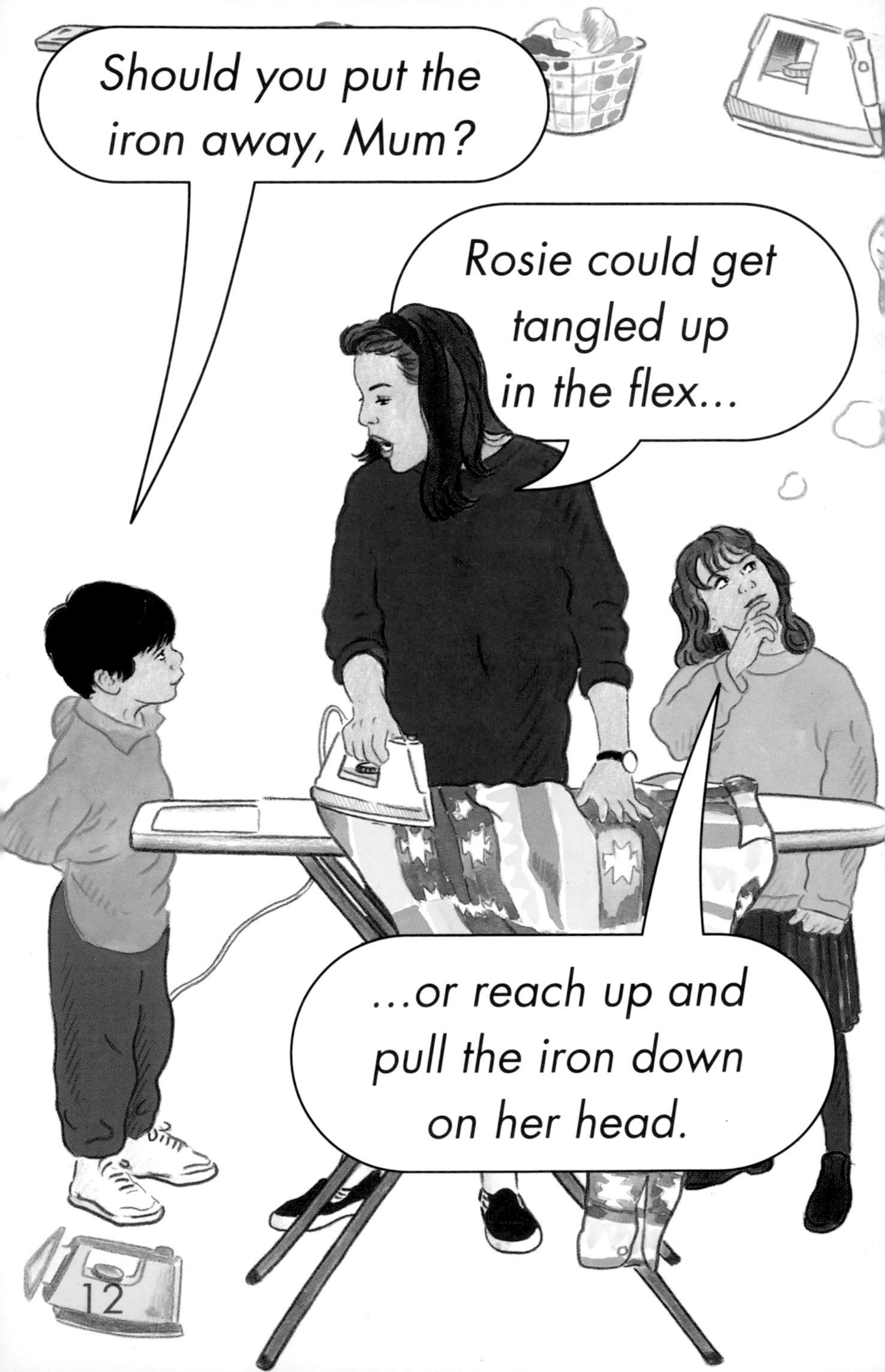
Should you put the iron away, Mum?
Rosie could get tangled up in the flex...
...or reach up and pull the iron down on her head.

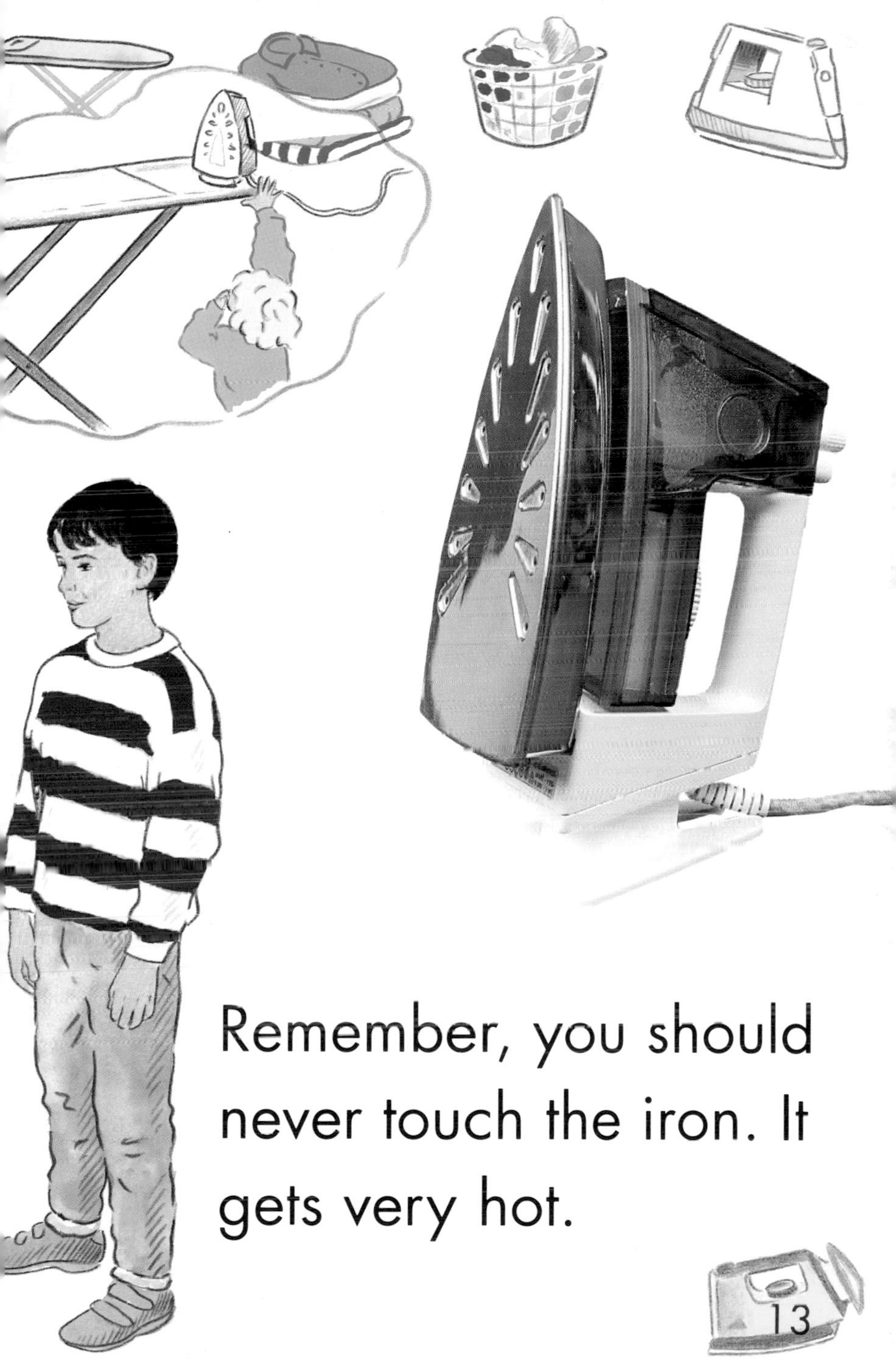

Remember, you should never touch the iron. It gets very hot.

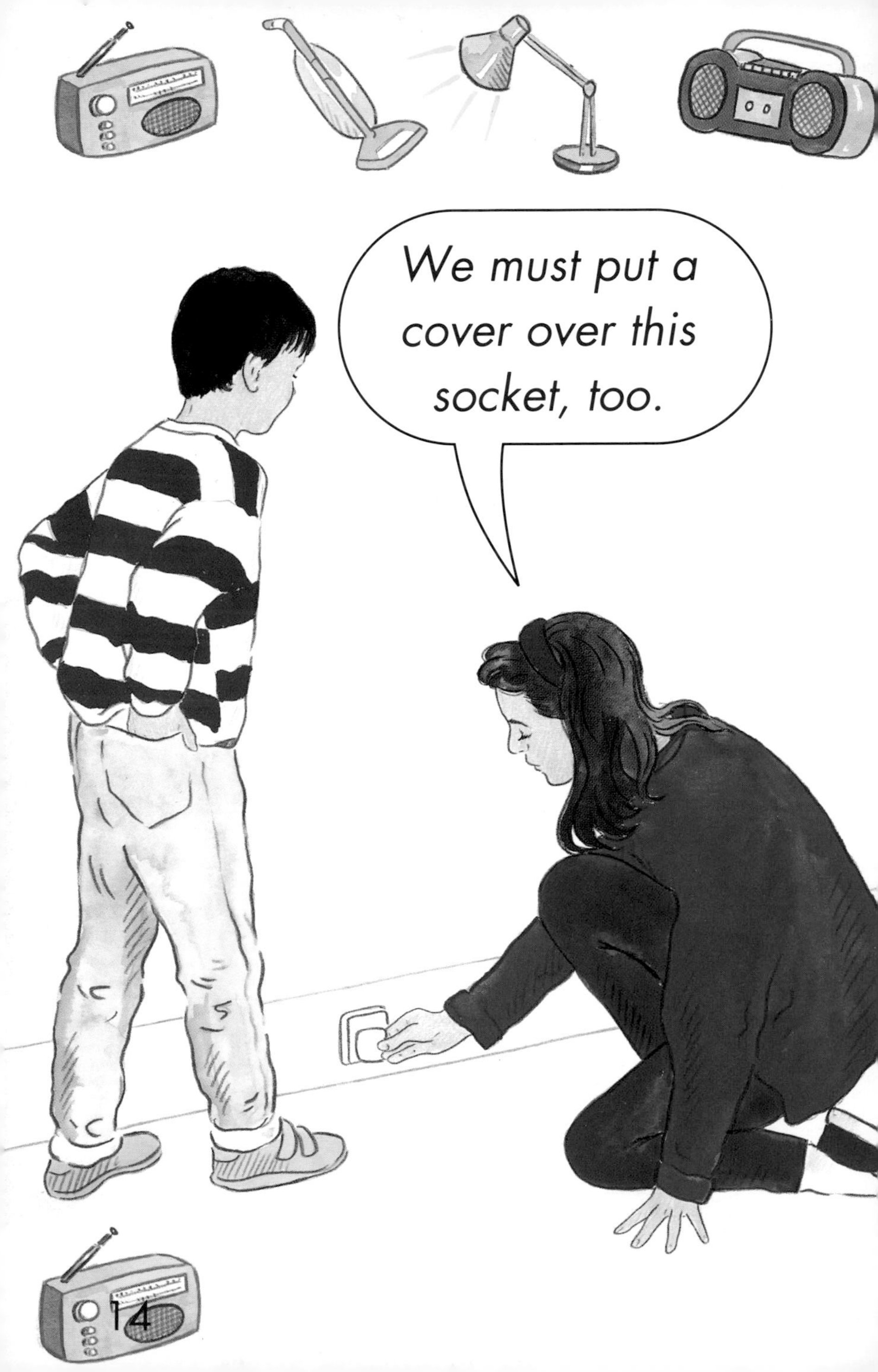
We must put a cover over this socket, too.

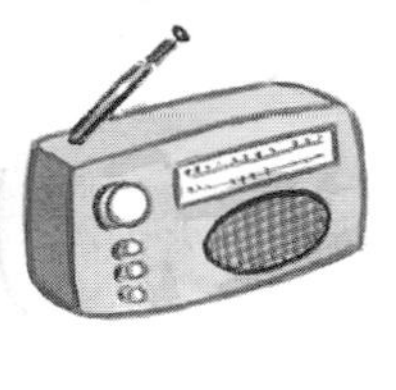

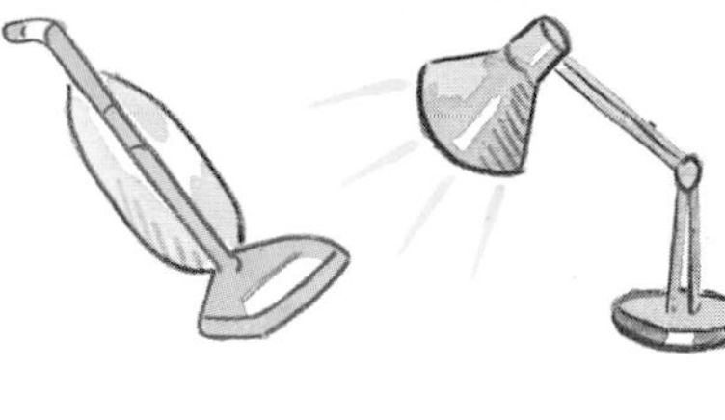

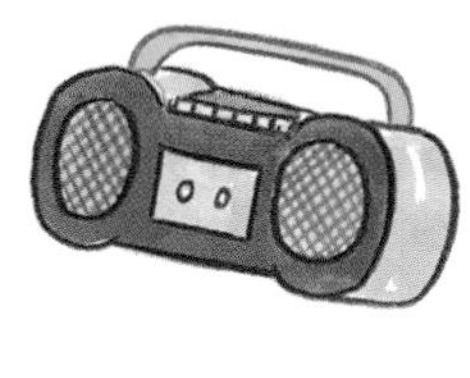

Electric sockets are dangerous and you should never touch them.

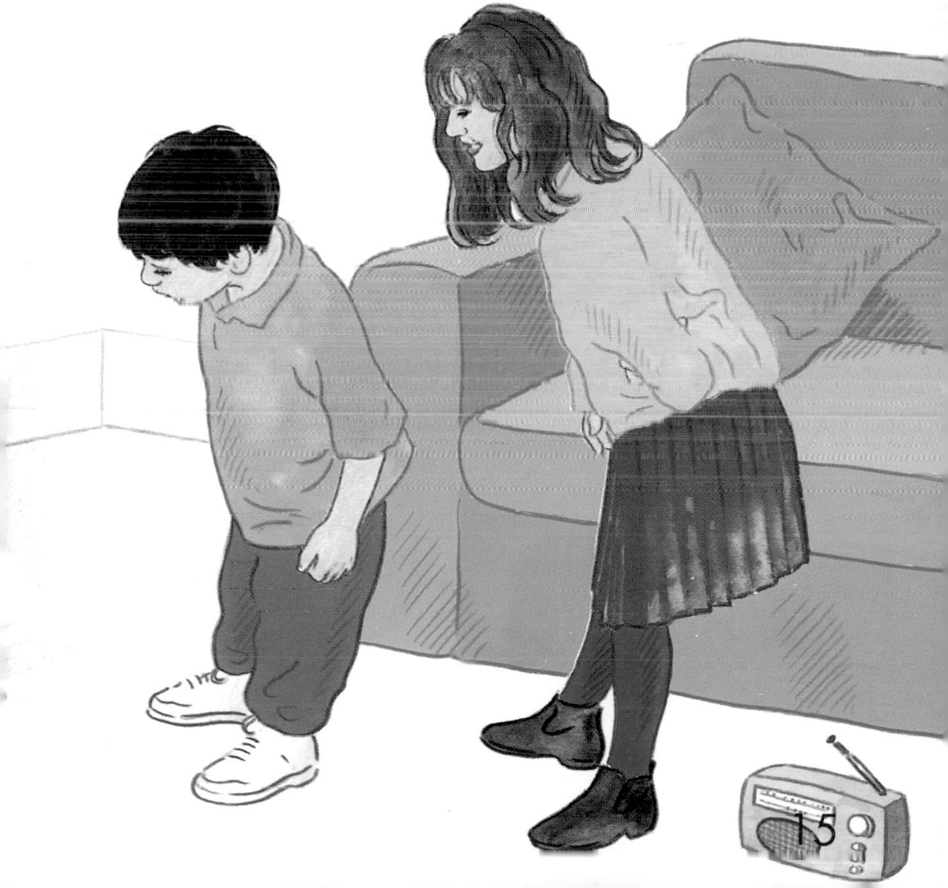

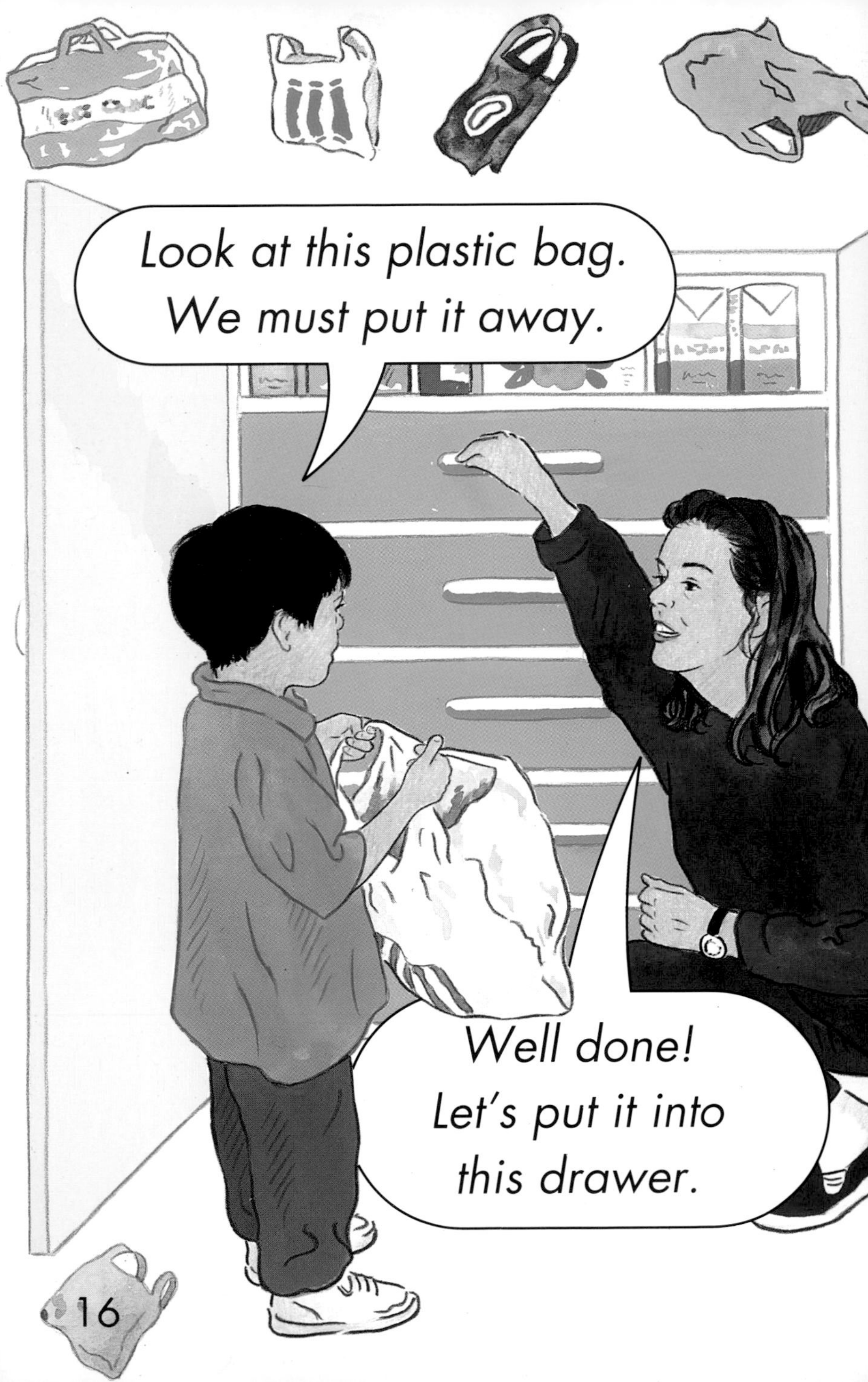
Look at this plastic bag.
We must put it away.
Well done!
Let's put it into
this drawer.

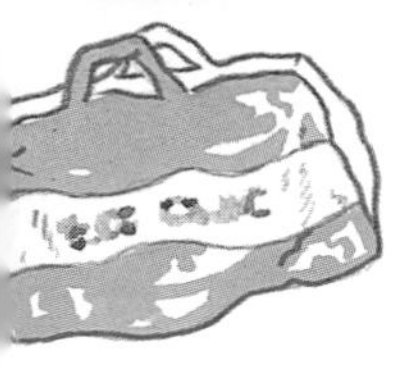
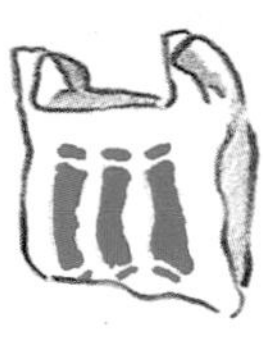
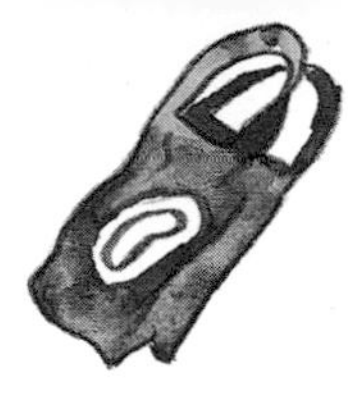
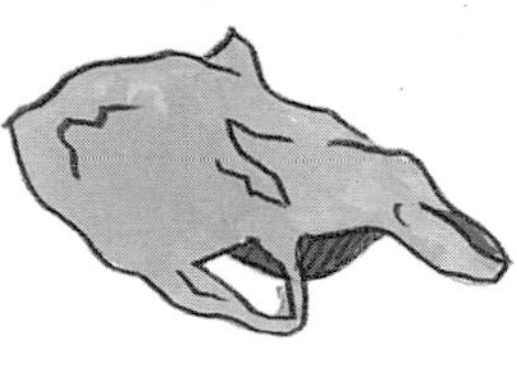

Plastic bags are dangerous. Rosie could put one over her head and then she wouldn't be able to breathe.

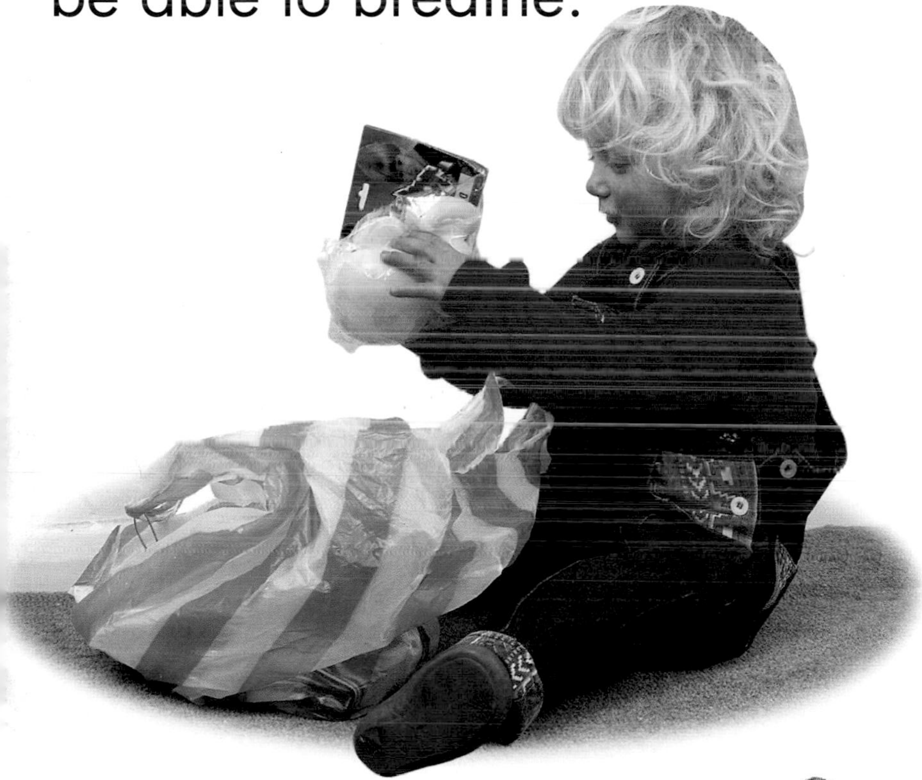

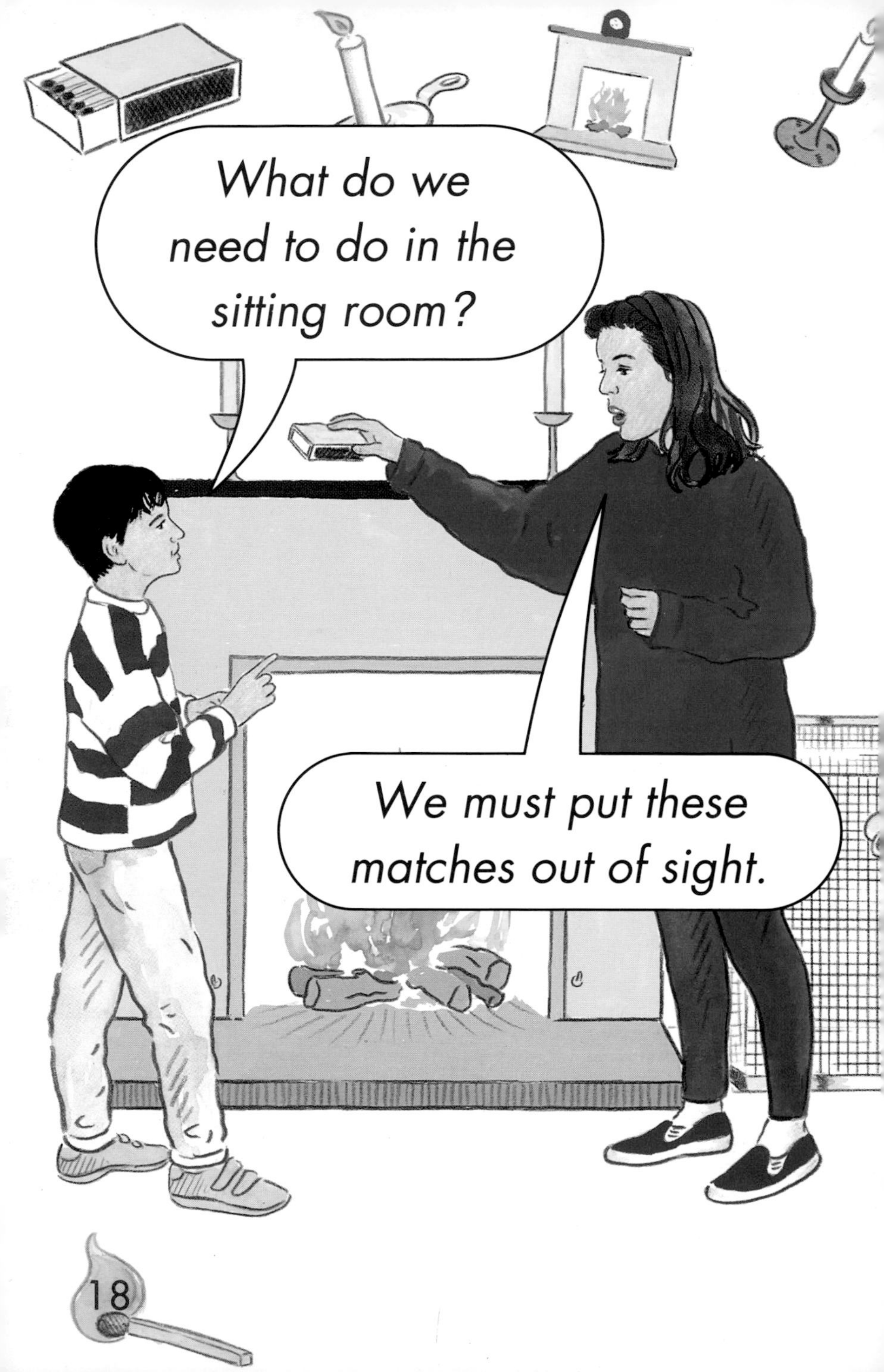
What do we need to do in the sitting room?
We must put these matches out of sight.

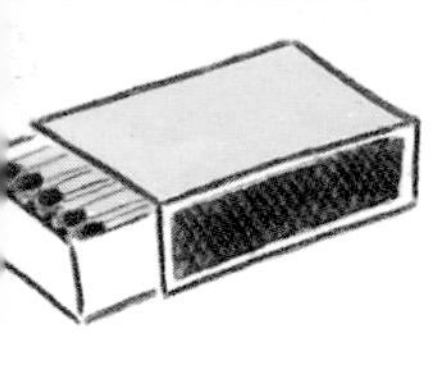
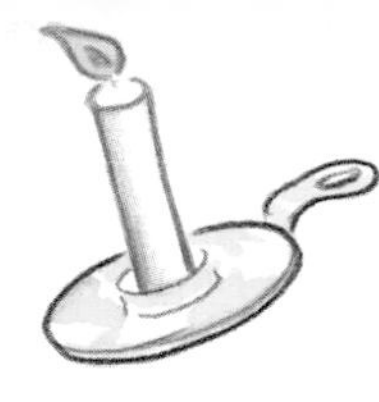
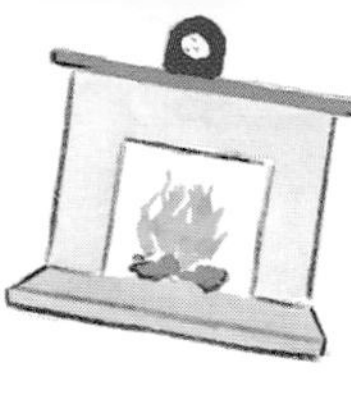
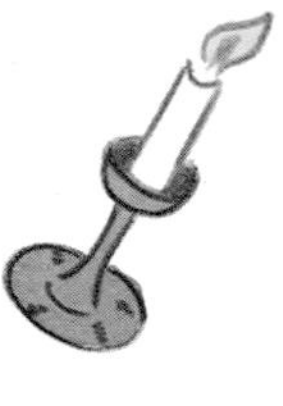

You should never play with matches. It's easy to burn yourself or start a fire.

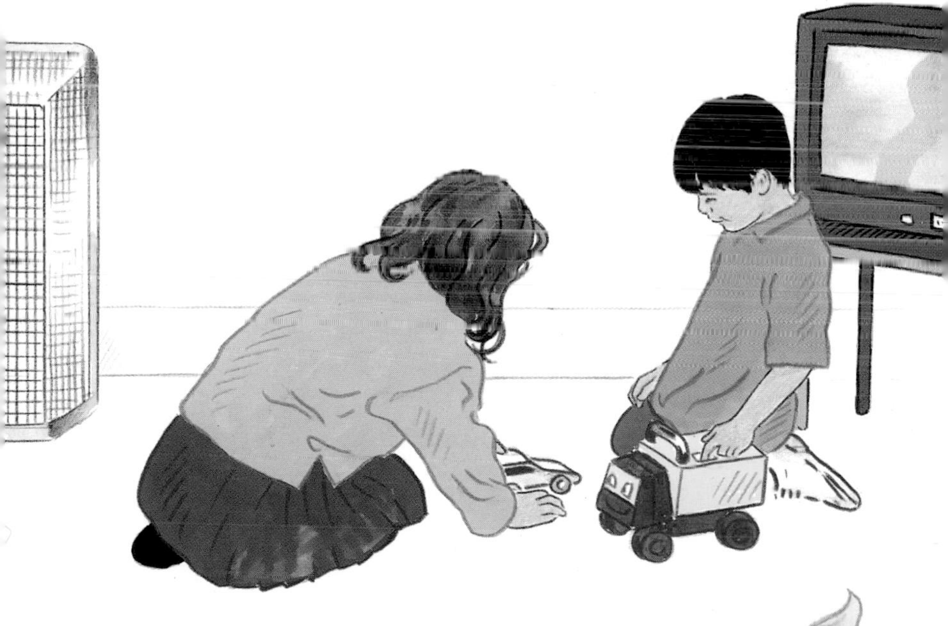

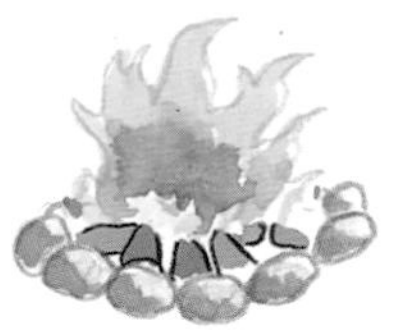
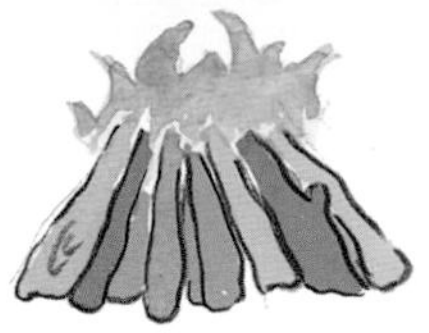
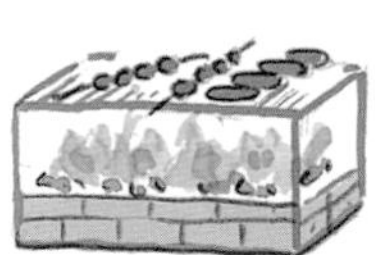
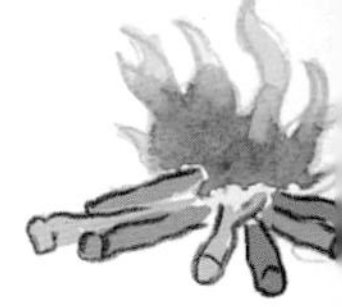

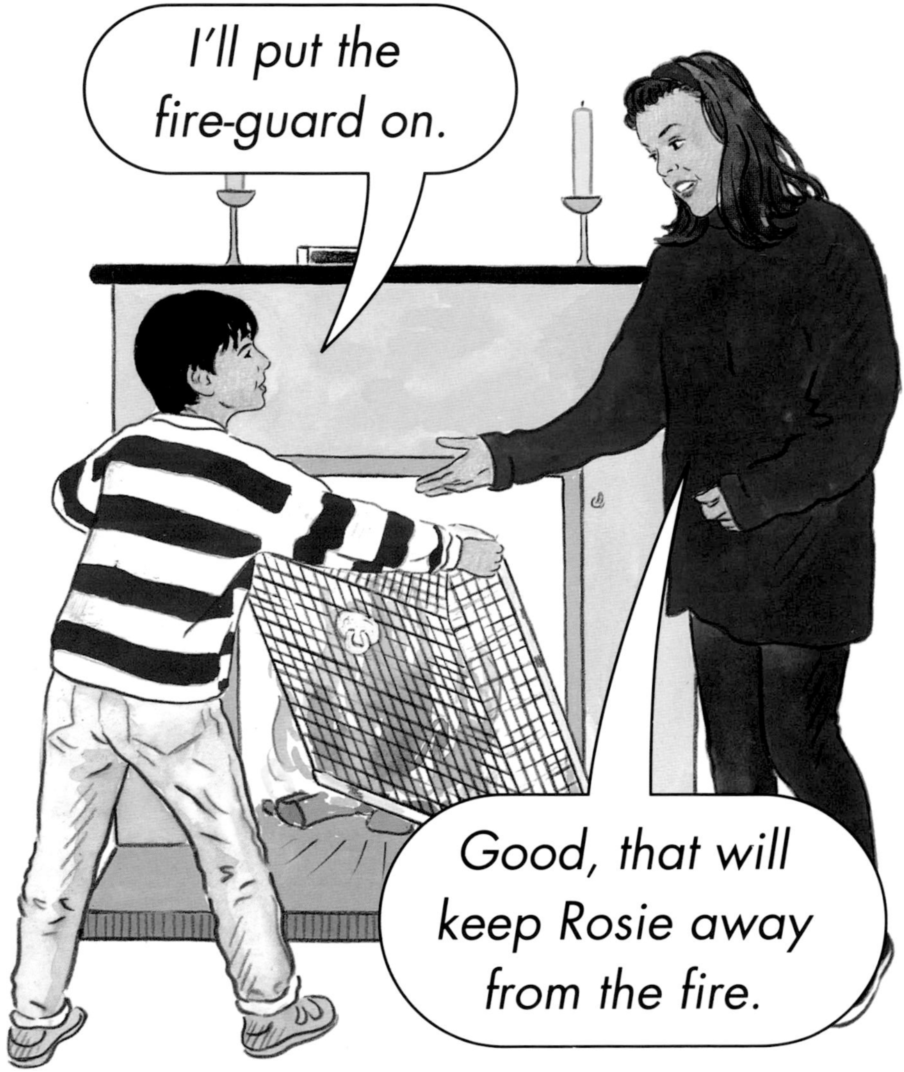

I'll put the fire-guard on.

Good, that will keep Rosie away from the fire.

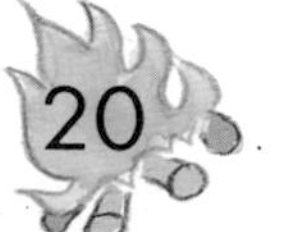

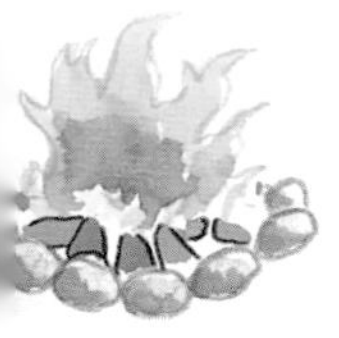 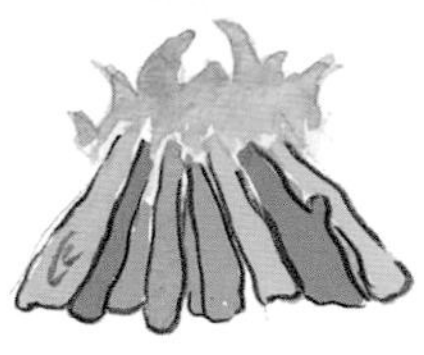 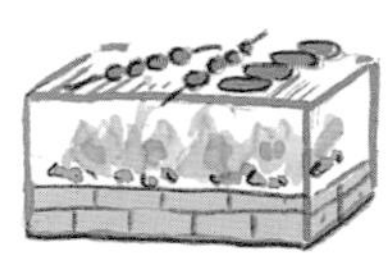 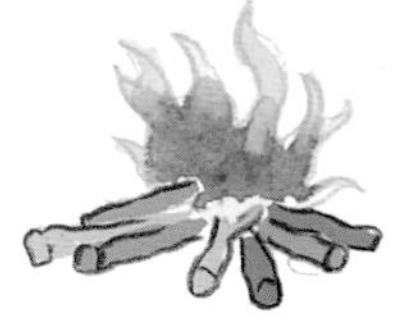

Never stand or sit too close to the fire. You could get burnt.

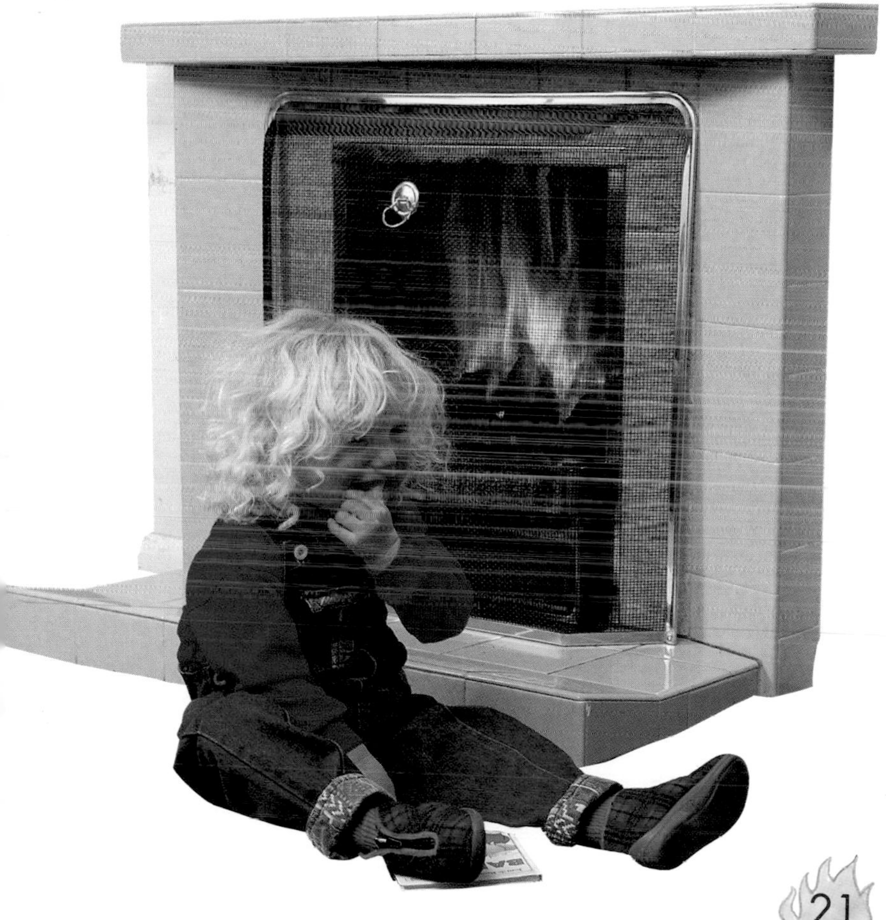

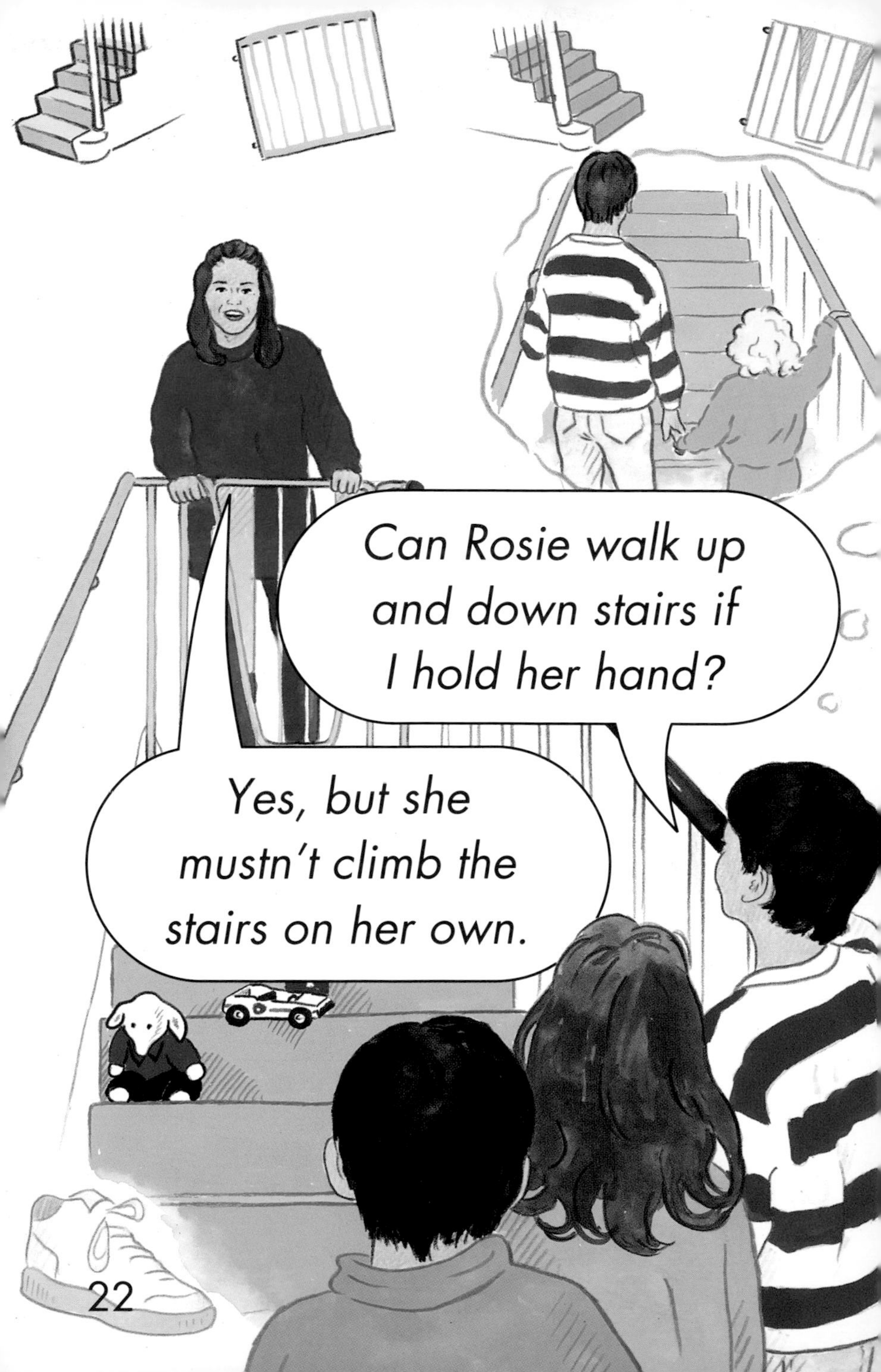
Can Rosie walk up and down stairs if I hold her hand?
Yes, but she mustn't climb the stairs on her own.

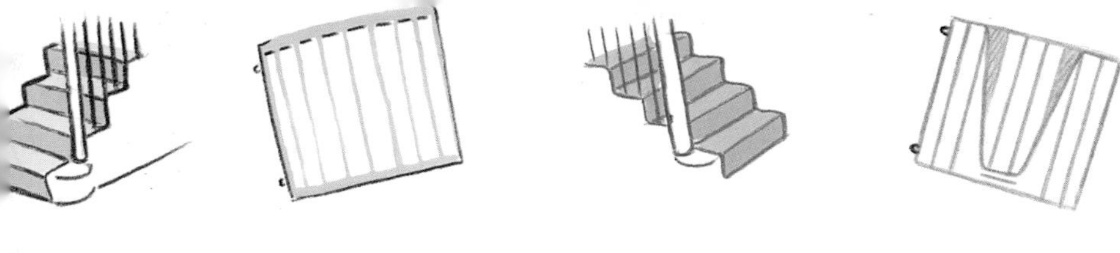

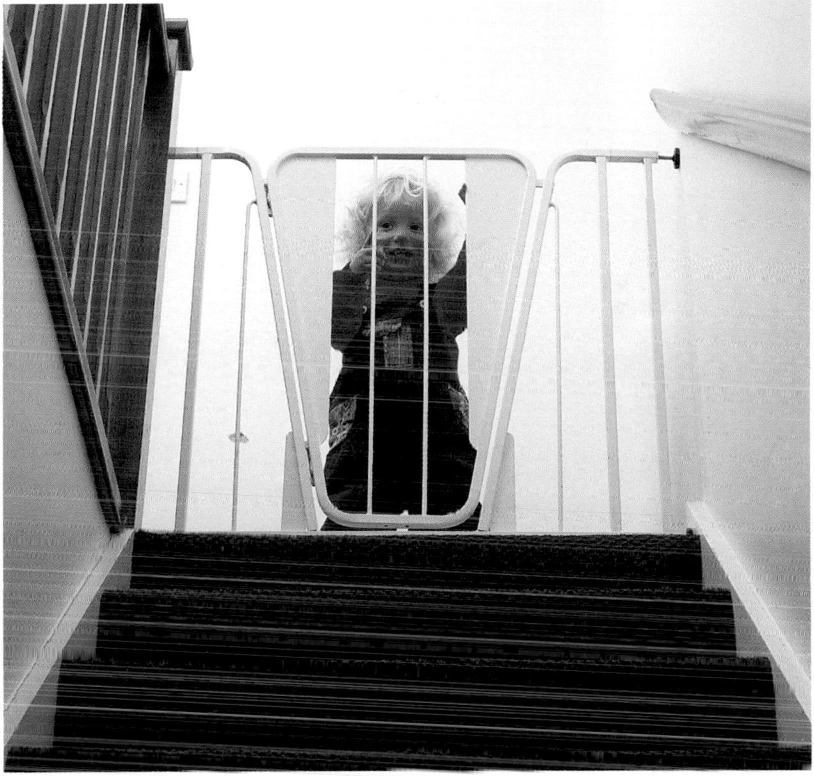

Never leave anything on the stairs. You could trip over and hurt yourself.

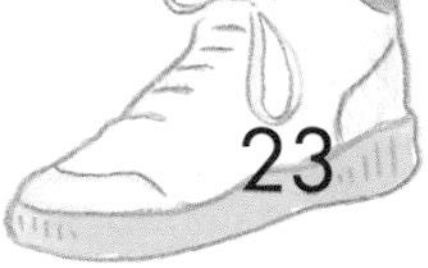

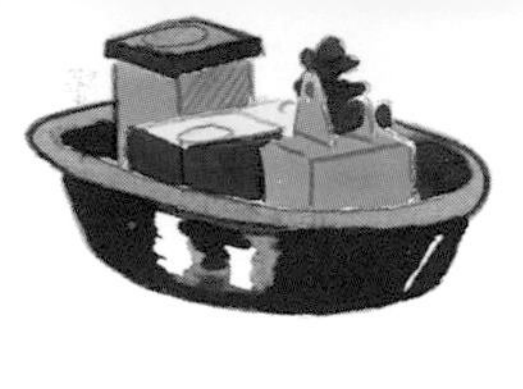

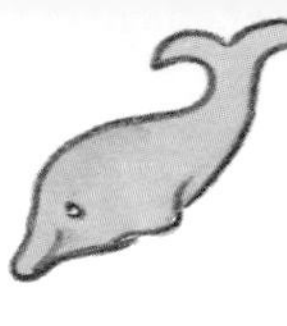

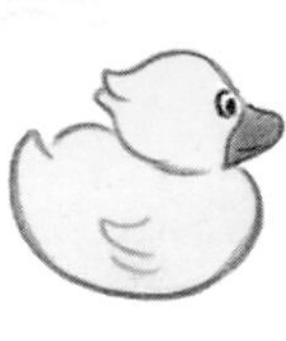

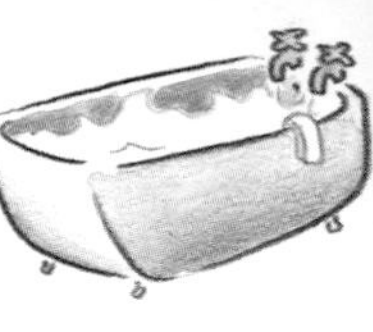

Rosie will want a bath before she goes to bed.

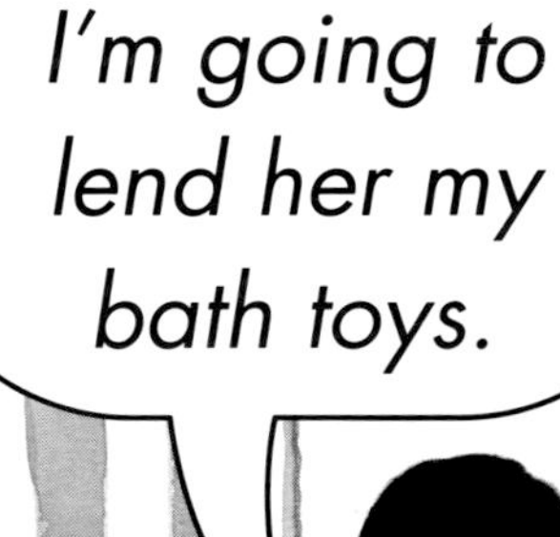

I'm going to lend her my bath toys.

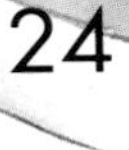

We must put all of these cleaning liquids out of reach.

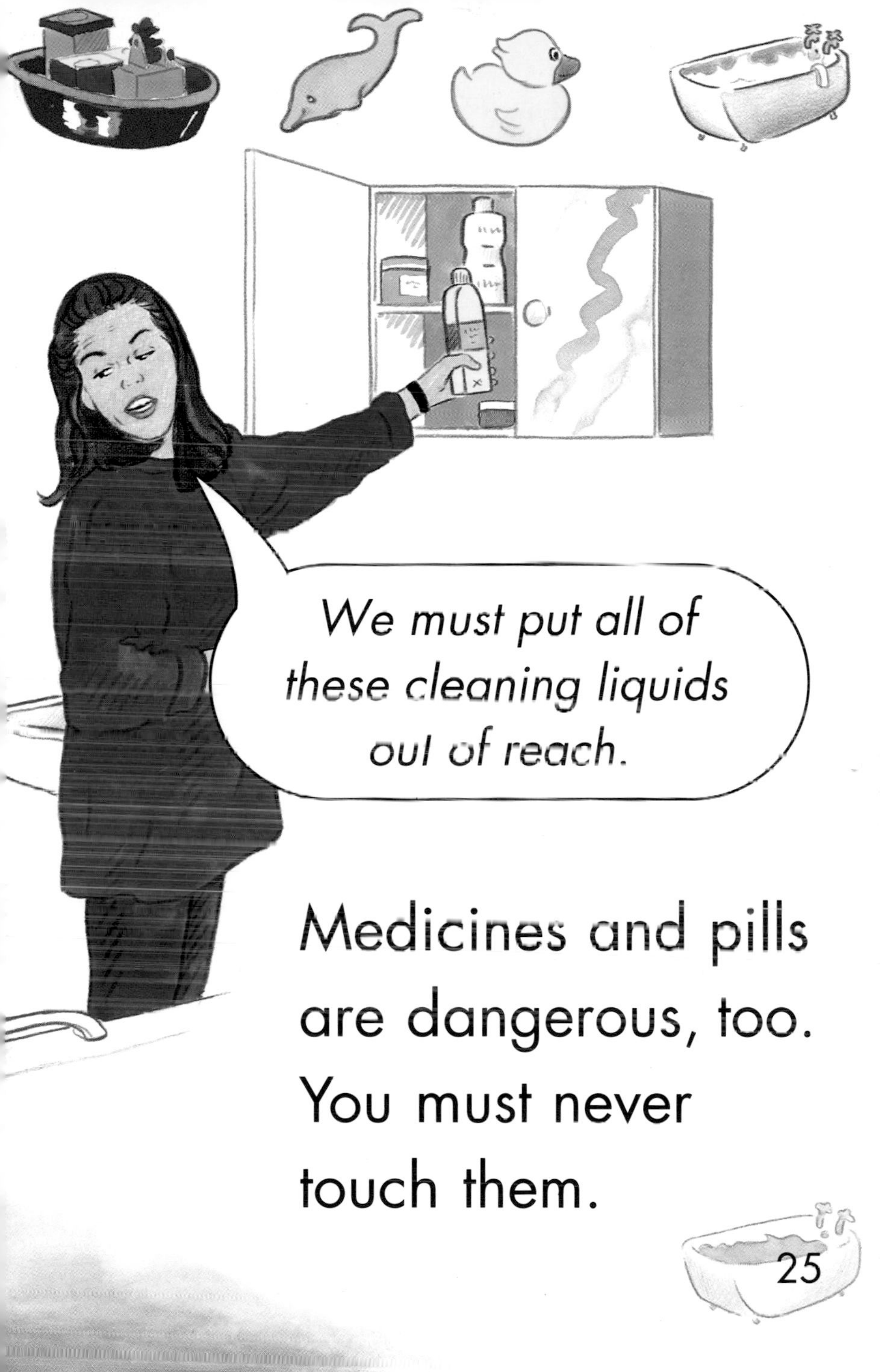

Medicines and pills are dangerous, too. You must never touch them.

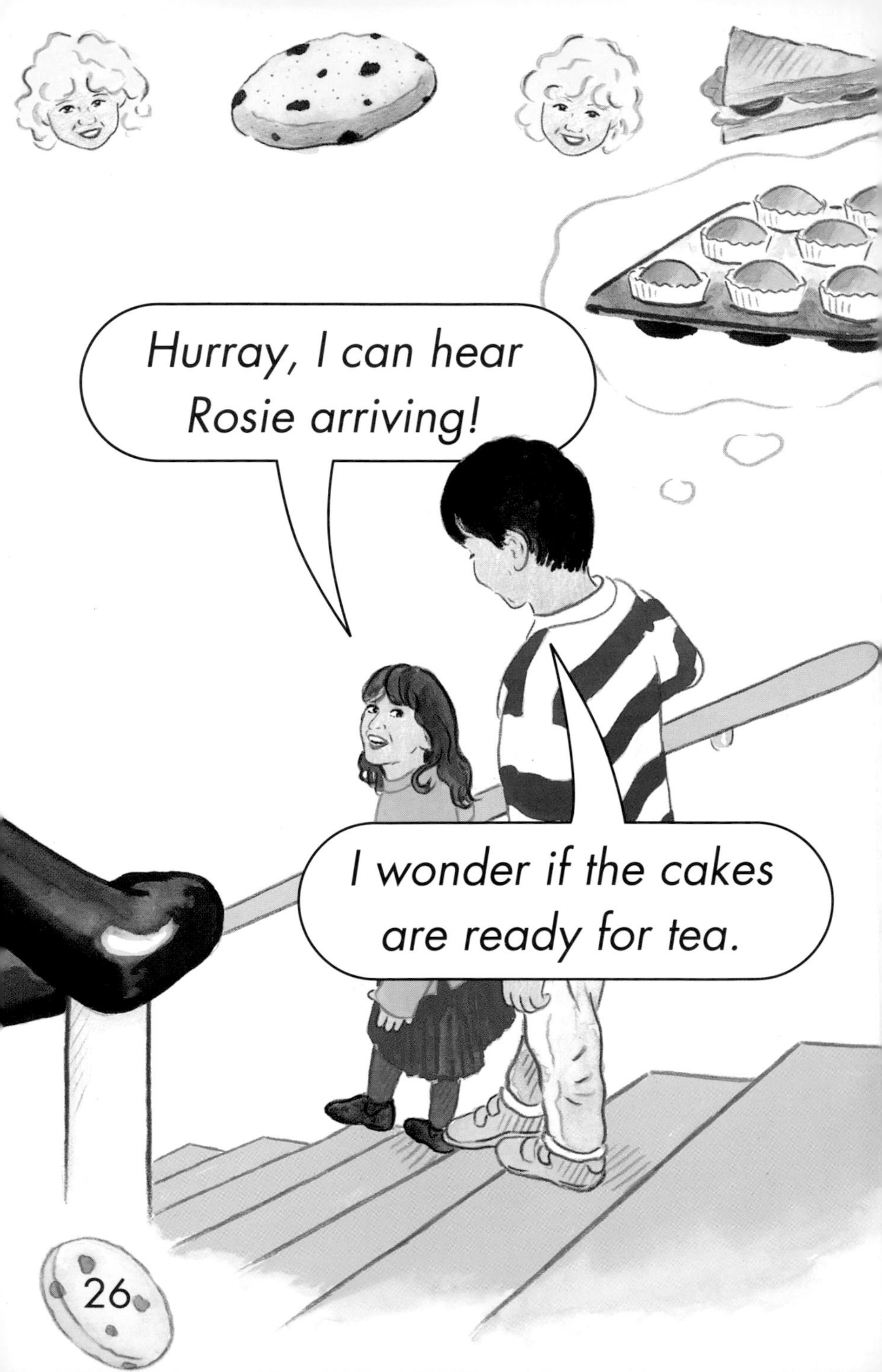
Hurray, I can hear Rosie arriving!
I wonder if the cakes are ready for tea.

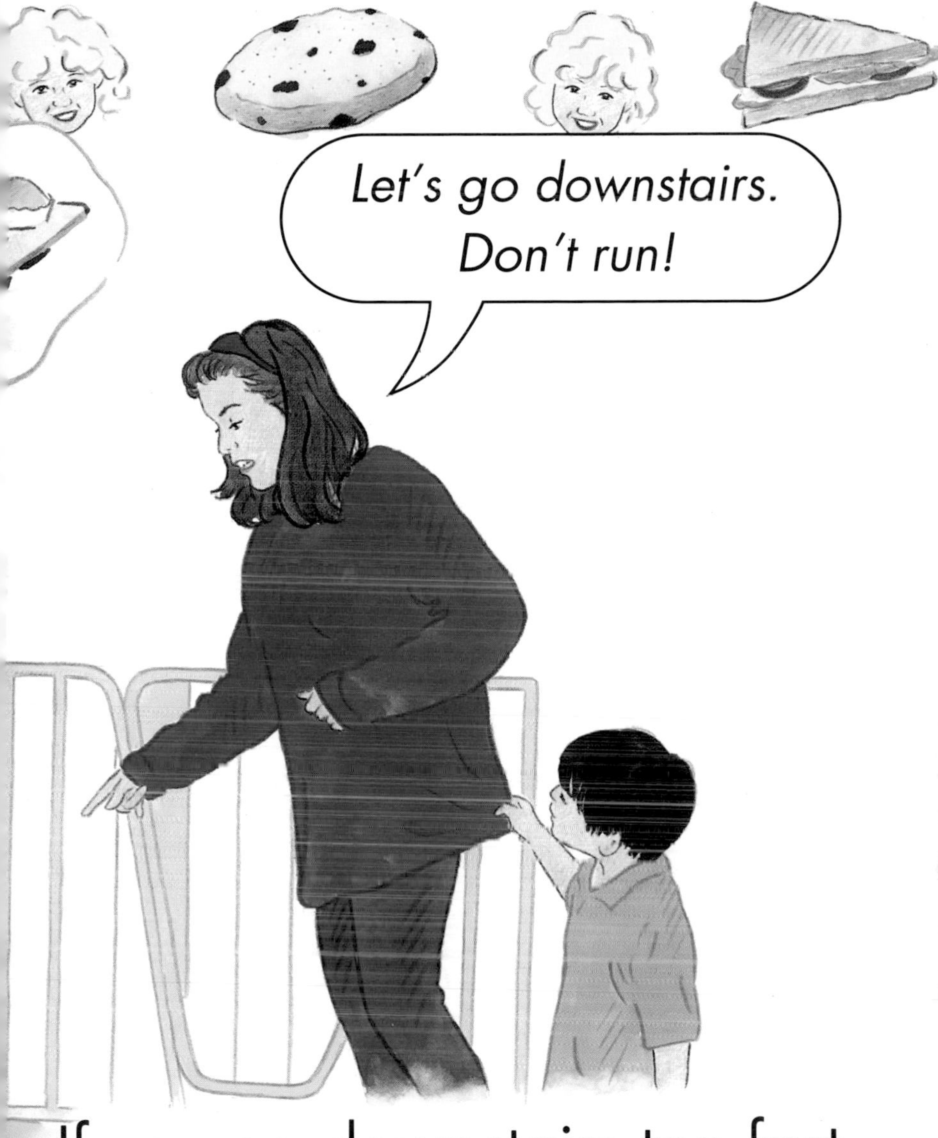

If you go downstairs too fast you could fall.

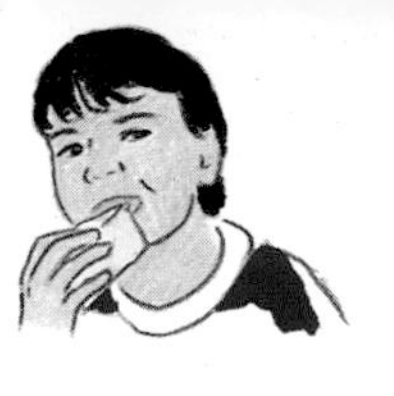
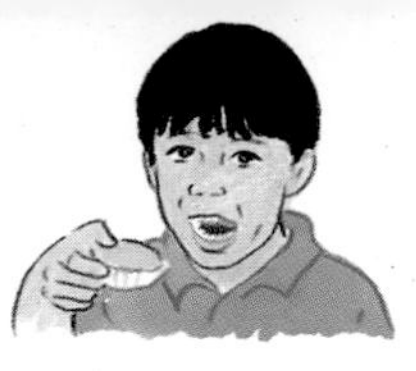
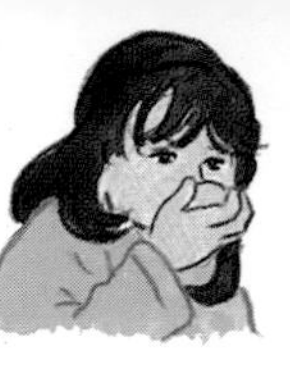
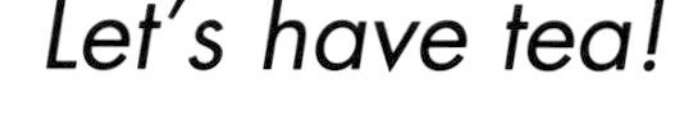
Let's have tea!
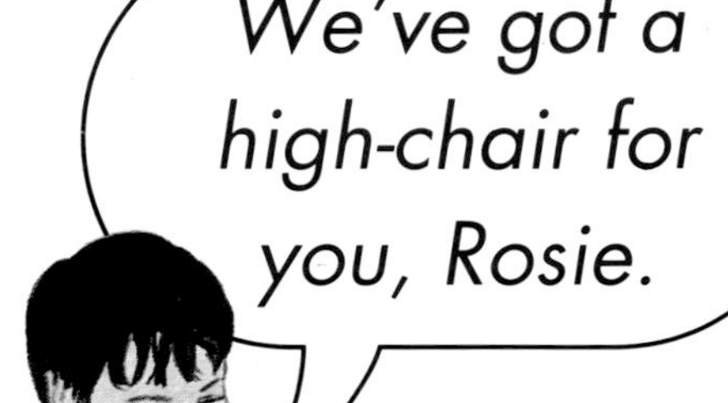
We've got a
high-chair for
you, Rosie.
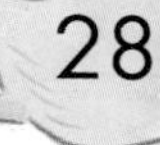

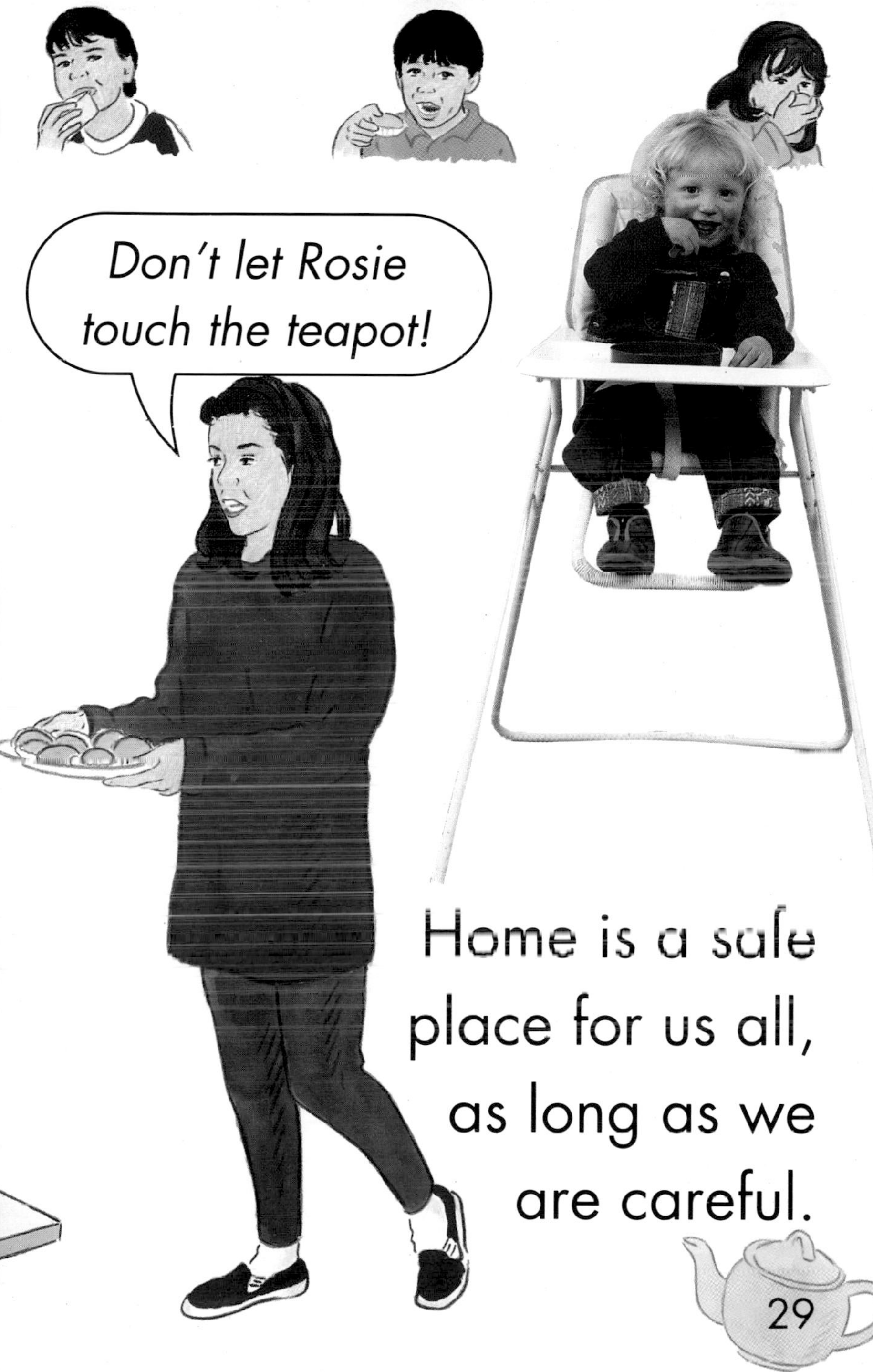

Home is a safe
place for us all,
as long as we
are careful.

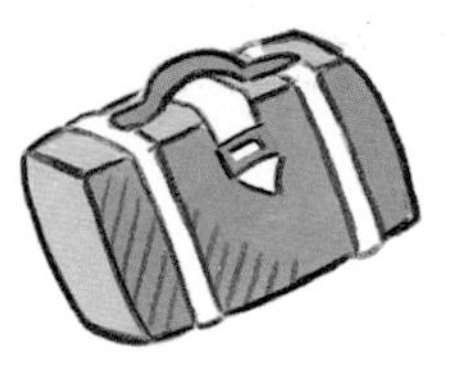 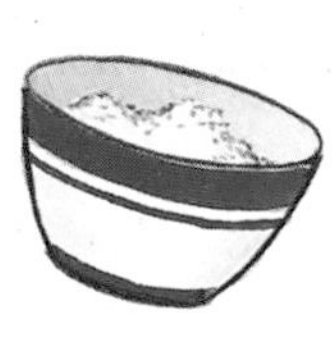 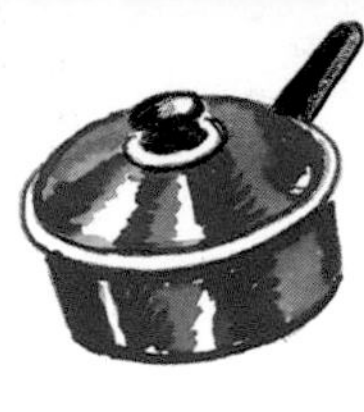 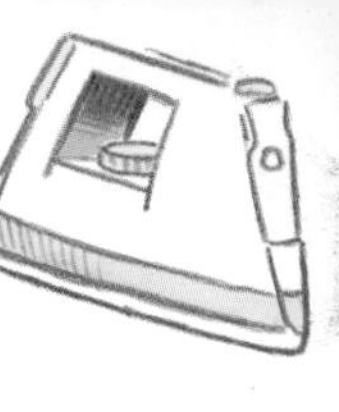

Here is a room in someone's home. What would you do to make it safe for a young child?

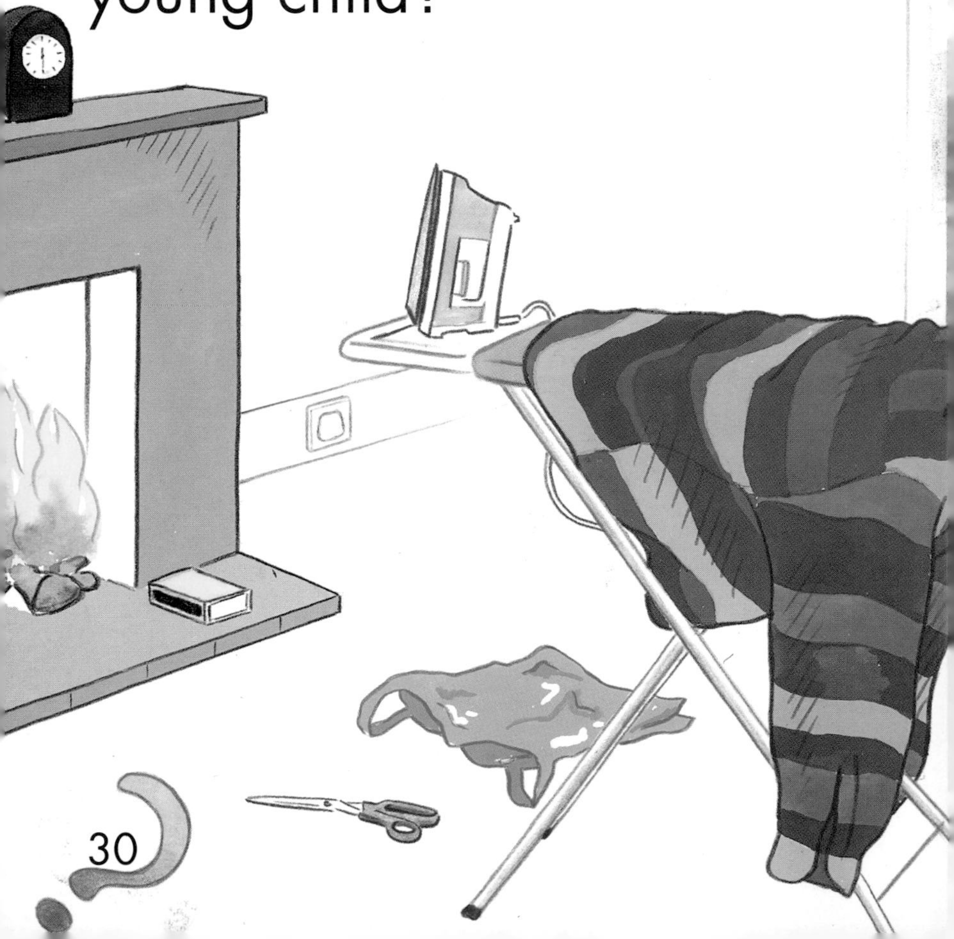